# NAVIGATING VAGINAL CANCER WITH CONFIDENCE AND CARE



Empowering Insights And Strategies For Confronting Vaginal Health Challenges For Vibrant Healing

## DR. WESLEY IAN

# DISCLAIMER

The information in this book is not meant to replace professional medical advice, diagnosis, or treatment; rather, it is meant mainly for general informational reasons. If you have any questions about a medical problem, you should always consult your doctor or another trained health expert. Don't ever discount expert medical advice or put off getting it because of something you've read in this book.

Any negative effects or repercussions arising from the usage of the material provided herein are not the responsibility of the book's author or publisher. It should be noted by readers that the material in this book is not all-inclusive and might not address every facet of the subject. Furthermore, new research may have an impact on how health concerns are understood or treated because medical knowledge is always changing.

No particular test, treatment, method, or product mentioned in this book is endorsed or promoted by the author or publisher. The reader assumes all risk associated with using the information included in this book.

Before making any big decisions regarding your health, it's crucial to speak with a licensed healthcare provider. The relationship between a patient and their healthcare practitioner should not be replaced by this book, nor is it meant to offer medical advice.

The opinions presented in this book are the author's and may not necessarily represent those of the publisher. Any errors, omissions, or inaccuracies in the information in this book are not the responsibility of the author or publisher.

It is recommended that readers independently confirm any information contained in this book and speak with a healthcare provider about their specific medical needs and state of health.

# TABLE OF CONTENTS

# ABOUT THE BOOK

For those coping with the difficulties of vaginal cancer, "Navigating Vaginal Cancer with Confidence and Care" is an invaluable resource. It offers thorough insights into the illness and equips readers to handle the complexities of diagnosis, treatment, emotional health, and survivorship. With this basic knowledge, readers will be able to better understand the subtleties of the illness and make well-informed decisions about their healthcare path.

The book dives into the diagnostic environment, providing a thorough examination of screening, early detection, diagnostic techniques, and cancer staging. Readers are given the tools to actively participate in their treatment plans by this section, which demystifies the technical components of the diagnostic procedure and assists in interpreting test results. The book moves smoothly, where it discusses various treatment choices and recommends a multidisciplinary strategy that includes immunotherapy, hormone therapy, radiation therapy, chemotherapy, and surgery. With the help of this thorough summary, patients can feel more in control of their treatment choices and can have educated conversations with their medical team.

Understanding the significant influence that emotional health has on the cancer journey, focuses on building a strong support network. It offers helpful advice on establishing a support system, having productive conversations with loved ones, and working with medical specialists. It delves deeper into the psychological difficulties that accompany receiving a cancer diagnosis. It provides coping mechanisms for fear, worry, and sadness while encouraging optimism and hope.

The book delves into lifestyle and wellness factors, expanding its scope beyond medical procedures. Integrative therapies, exercise, diet, and managing the side effects of therapy are just a few of the topics that highlight the comprehensive approach to cancer care.

# CHAPTER ONE

## INTRODUCTION TO VAGINAL CANCER

### KNOWING ABOUT CERVICAL CANCER

The tissues of the vagina, the muscular tube that connects the cervix (the bottom part of the uterus) to the external genitalia, are affected by vaginal cancer, an uncommon but dangerous medical illness. This type of cancer can present with many different symptoms, making diagnosis and therapy extremely difficult. It is crucial to explore all of the aspects of vaginal cancer, such as its description, types, underlying causes, associated risk factors, and the telltale signs and symptoms that may suggest its presence, to fully understand the complexities surrounding this condition.

### VAGINAL CANCER: WHAT IS IT?

One kind of cancer that starts in the vaginal cells is called vaginal cancer. A vital component of the female reproductive system, the vagina is essential to menstruation, childbirth, and sexual activity. Vaginal cancer can develop as a result of aberrant cells inside the vaginal walls growing out of control and developing into a tumor.

Despite being less common than other forms of cancer, this illness warrants attention because it may hurt a woman's general health and well-being.

## VAGINAL CANCER TYPES

Vaginal cancer is not a single disease; rather, it is a group of diseases, each with its special traits and effects. The two most common types are adenocarcinoma, which starts in the glandular cells, and squamous cell carcinoma, which develops from the thin, flat cells covering the surface of the vagina. Sarcoma, clear cell carcinoma, and melanoma are among the less frequent varieties. Comprehending these variances is essential to customizing efficacious therapeutic approaches and ensuring optimal patient outcomes.

# REASONS AND DANGER ELEMENTS

Determining the precise causes of vaginal cancer is still difficult since a complex interaction of genetic, environmental, and lifestyle variables frequently play a role. A known risk factor is ongoing infection with specific strains of the human papillomavirus (HPV), which is linked to most vaginal malignancies. A history of cervical cancer, exposure to diethylstilbestrol (DES) before delivery, smoking, and compromised immune function are other variables that may increase the risk. Determining these contributing factors is essential to creating targeted interventions and preventative actions for more vulnerable individuals.

## SYMPTOMS AND INDICATIONS

For early detection and better treatment outcomes, it is essential to recognize the telltale signs and symptoms of vaginal cancer. Unusual vaginal bleeding, pain during sexual activity, pelvic pain unrelated to menstruation, and a visible lump or tumor in the vagina are common indicators.

The vagueness of these symptoms makes it difficult to instantly link them to vaginal cancer, which emphasizes the significance of routine gynecological exams and candid communication between patients and medical professionals. Early detection of these warning indicators may help to speed up medical action and improve the prognosis for recovery and treatment.

Learning about the nuances of vaginal cancer entails investigating everything from its description and types to its underlying causes, related risk factors, and the most important indications and symptoms that indicate the disease's existence. Advances in medical research have led to an evolution of information regarding vaginal cancer, which has resulted in improved diagnostic techniques, tailored therapy, and better outcomes for individuals afflicted with this difficult ailment.

# CHAPTER TWO

## RECOGNITION AND SEQUENCING

## EARLY DETECTION AND SCREENING

To diagnose cancers at an early, more manageable stage, screening and early detection are essential to the efficient therapy of cancer. The process of screening entails the methodical use of tests or examinations to find cancer in people who may not yet exhibit symptoms. These tests are frequently given to people who fall into particular age ranges or who have particular risk factors. Pap smears for cervical cancer, colonoscopies for colorectal cancer, and mammograms for breast cancer are a few examples of frequently used screening techniques.

On the other hand, early detection entails identifying cancer while it is still confined and has not yet spread. Early identification is important since it might lead to less aggressive treatment options and better results.

# PROCEDURES FOR DIAGNOSIS

Confirming the existence of cancer following a positive screening or in cases where symptoms are apparent requires the use of diagnostic methods. The kind, location, and degree of cancer are all determined using a variety of diagnostic instruments and methods. Imaging tests, which include CT, MRI, PET, and X-rays, offer comprehensive visual data regarding the tumor's location in adjacent tissues. A biopsy is an essential diagnostic technique that includes taking a tiny sample of tissue from the suspected malignant spot and examining it under a microscope. This makes it possible for pathologists to determine the cancer's type and evaluate its attributes, such as aggressiveness and potential for metastasis.

## SETTING UP THE MALIGNANCY

Determining the size, location, and if the cancer has progressed to surrounding or distant organs is known as staging, and it is a crucial step in the diagnosis of cancer. The cancer's stage influences therapy choices and offers important prognostic data. For staging purposes, the TNM (Tumor, Node, and Metastasis) method is frequently employed. In this system, T stands for the size of the original tumor, N for the involvement of neighboring lymph nodes, and M for the existence of distant metastases. Roman numerals are commonly used to represent the stages, which range from 0 (in situ or localized) to IV (advanced or metastatic). Oncologists can better customize treatment approaches using staging by taking into account the unique features of the cancer and how it is progressing.

## ANALYZING TEST FINDINGS

A crucial part of the diagnosis procedure is interpreting test results, which calls for cooperation between oncologists, radiologists, and pathologists among other medical specialists. The outcomes of pathology reports and imaging studies offer important details regarding the type and features of the malignancy. To determine the kind, grade, and other molecular indicators of cancer that may impact treatment choices, pathologists examine biopsy specimens. Radiologists analyze imaging data to ascertain the tumor's location, size, and extent of spread. Through cooperative analysis of these data, cancer specialists can decide on the best course of treatment by considering the unique features of each patient's malignancy as well as their general health. Accurate interpretation and a thorough comprehension of the diagnostic findings depend on clear communication and multidisciplinary teamwork.

# CHAPTER THREE
## OPTIONS FOR TREATMENT
### MULTIDISCIPLINARY METHOD

In the field of cancer care in particular, the multidisciplinary approach to therapy has emerged as a key component in the management of many medical problems. Several medical specialists work together as part of this holistic approach to provide a thorough and individualized treatment plan for the patient. A multidisciplinary team in the context of cancer usually consists of pathologists, radiologists, surgeons, oncologists, and other medical specialists.

This strategy has the advantage of being able to handle the intricacy of cancer by taking into account not only the tumor itself but also its possible effects on many bodily systems. The multidisciplinary approach aims to improve patient care, optimize treatment outcomes, and raise the overall quality of life both during and after treatment by combining diverse medical views.

# OPTIONS FOR SURGERY

For many different kinds of malignancies, surgery is still a basic and frequently the first course of treatment. To eradicate or lessen the malignant growth, tumors or impacted tissues must be removed. Surgical therapies, contingent on the type, location, and size of the tumor, can vary from minimally invasive procedures, such as laparoscopy, to more involved open surgeries. In addition to removing the obvious tumor, surgery aims to evaluate and maybe remove adjacent lymph nodes to ascertain the full degree of the illness. Surgery is becoming a more successful and well-tolerated therapeutic option because of improvements in surgical procedures, such as robotic-assisted surgery, which have increased precision and shortened recovery times for many patients.

## RADIATION TREATMENT

High radiation doses are used in radiation therapy, commonly referred to as radiotherapy, to target and kill cancer cells. When the tumor is confined and can be carefully targeted, this therapeutic approach is especially effective. Radiation therapy can be applied internally by putting radioactive sources close to or inside the tumor, or externally by utilizing devices that target radiation beams at the affected area. The intention is to harm cancer cells' DNA so that it can't divide and proliferate. Depending on the particulars of the malignancy, radiation therapy may be utilized as a stand-alone treatment or in conjunction with other treatments like surgery or chemotherapy.

## CHEMOTHERAPY

Drugs are used in chemotherapy to either kill or stop the growth of rapidly proliferating cells, such as cancer cells. These medications can be injected or taken orally, and they work by traveling throughout the body to target the main tumor as well as any possible metastases.

Chemotherapy targets fast-dividing cells, a hallmark of cancer, even though it is a systemic treatment that affects all of the body's cells. Because it affects healthy cells, chemotherapy can have side effects, but because of developments in supportive care and chemotherapy regimens, tolerance has improved for many patients. Chemotherapy is frequently used in combination with other therapies to manage cancer more thoroughly and effectively.

## IMMUNOTHERAPY

Using the body's immune system to identify and combat cancer cells, immunotherapy is a new method of treating cancer. Immunotherapy boosts the immune system to improve its capacity to recognize and eliminate cancer cells, in contrast to conventional treatments that target cancer cells directly.

There are other immunotherapy approaches, such as cancer vaccines, adoptive cell treatments, and immune checkpoint inhibitors. Immunotherapy offers new hope to patients, especially those with advanced or metastatic disease, and has been incorporated into standard treatment regimens due to its exceptional efficacy in treating some cancers.

# HORMONE TREATMENT

Endocrine therapy, or hormone therapy, is a focused therapeutic method frequently used for hormone-sensitive malignancies, including prostate and breast cancers. Hormones like testosterone and estrogen have an impact on certain malignancies and encourage their growth. The way hormone treatment functions is by either preventing these hormones from being produced or by interfering with their function. For instance, aromatase inhibitors or selective estrogen receptor modulators (SERMs) may be used as part of hormone therapy for breast cancer. Similar to this, androgen restriction therapy lowers testosterone levels in patients with prostate cancer. The use of hormone therapy as an adjuvant or in situations when surgery or radiation therapy may not be enough to manage the disease highlights the significance of tailored and focused techniques in the treatment of cancer.

# CHAPTER FOUR

## PUTTING TOGETHER YOUR SUPPORT GROUP

### CREATING A HELPFUL NETWORK

Building a network of support is essential to developing resilience and emotional health. It entails developing deep relationships with people who can provide support, empathy, and a sense of belonging. A range of ties, such as those with family, friends, coworkers, and mentors, may be included in this network. Creating a network of support involves giving as well as receiving support to create a mutually advantageous system of support and encouragement.

### SPEAKING WITH FRIENDS AND FAMILY

Having good connections and getting the support you need during trying times depend on having effective communication with family and friends. Honest and transparent communication facilitates the expression of wants, feelings, and worries and promotes a higher level of understanding between people. Not only can sharing experiences and feelings with those you love deepen the relationship, but it also helps them understand the difficulties you confront. This dialogue emphasizes the value of emotional connection by creating a supportive environment where people feel heard, respected, and cared for.

## INCLUDING MEDICAL EXPERTS

In some circumstances, consulting with medical professionals is essential for complete support. These experts, who include physicians, therapists, and counselors, have the training and experience necessary to offer specialized support. Including medical specialists guarantees that patients have access to specialized advice, plans for treatment, and coping mechanisms. Working together, patients and healthcare professionals may address mental and physical health issues and develop a comprehensive strategy for well-being that goes beyond social networks.

# LOOKING FOR PSYCHOLOGICAL ASSISTANCE

A strong support system must include emotional assistance, which can be obtained in several ways. The main people you turn to for emotional support are usually friends and family since they can sympathize, encourage, and provide an ear.

Furthermore, support groups—both virtual and physical—offer a forum for people going through comparable struggles to exchange stories and perspectives.

Receiving focused emotional support through professional assistance, like therapy or counseling, is another efficient strategy. It is possible to build a robust foundation for enduring life's ups and downs by actively seeking support and acknowledging the significance of emotional well-being.

Creating a support network is a dynamic, continuous process that calls for focus, work, and a readiness to offer and accept assistance.

People can build a strong support system that enhances their general well-being by actively seeking emotional assistance, engaging healthcare experts when needed, establishing relationships within their networks, and keeping lines of communication open.

# CHAPTER FIVE

## HANDLING EMOTIONAL DIFFICULTIES

### MANAGING A DIAGNOSIS

Being diagnosed, especially if it concerns a medical problem, can be a very upsetting event on an emotional level. It frequently represents a major turning point in a person's life and necessitates a difficult transition process. In addition to negotiating the physical components of a diagnosis, coping with one's emotions also entails recognizing its emotional implications. People may struggle with a variety of feelings, such as loss, shock, and denial. Acknowledging the situation's reality and making adjustments to accommodate the changes it brings about are steps in the long process of acceptance.

### HANDLING ANXIETY AND FEAR

Anxiety and fear are normal reactions to uncertainty, and they can get worse when faced with difficulties like a health diagnosis or significant life events. It's critical to acknowledge and deal with these feelings in a healthy way. Creating coping skills, such as mindfulness and relaxation methods, can aid with anxiety management. Furthermore, getting help from loved ones, friends, or mental health specialists can be a great way to communicate worries and get direction. To progressively free oneself from the grasp of dread and anxiety and restore stability and control, it is essential to comprehend the causes of these emotions.

## DEALING WITH DEPRESSION

Getting a diagnosis or dealing with difficult situations in life might occasionally set off depressive symptoms. More than just melancholy, depression is a chronic feeling of pessimism and detachment from joy. A multimodal strategy that incorporates social support, professional intervention, and self-care is necessary to treat depression. Individual or group therapy can provide a secure setting for examining and resolving these feelings. Creating a network of support and doing happy, fulfilling things are two ways to help depression symptoms gradually go away. It's critical to recognize that asking for assistance is a show of perseverance and strength.

## DISCOVERING HAPPINESS AND HOPE

Finding optimism and hope becomes a transformative journey in the middle of other life hardships or emotional obstacles brought on by a diagnosis. Developing a good outlook entails purposefully reorienting one's attention to possibilities for personal development, resilience, and thankfulness. Having a positive viewpoint gives you a mental framework to help you navigate obstacles rather than making them less real. Making connections with people who have overcome comparable obstacles and discovered resilience might give one hope. Little triumphs and happy moments, however brief, add to the general feeling of optimism. Finding hope is ultimately a dynamic process that calls for constant introspection, flexibility, and a dedication to looking for the good things in life.

# CHAPTER SIX

## WAY OF LIFE AND HEALTH

### DIET AND NUTRITION

The foundation of a healthy lifestyle, these factors are essential to general well-being. The body gets the vital vitamins, minerals, and nutrients it needs from a well-balanced diet to perform at its best. It is important to pay attention to the quality of the food ingested as well as calorie counting.

A varied and vibrant meal full of nutritious grains, lean meats, fruits, and veggies improves digestion, boosts immunity, and increases energy.

Another part of developing a positive relationship with food is mindful eating. We may connect with our bodies' signals of hunger and fullness more deeply when we are mindful of what, when, and how much we consume. Including food that is locally and sustainably sourced in one's diet helps the environment as well as one's health.

# EXERCISE AND PHYSICAL ACTIVITY

A wellness-focused lifestyle must include regular physical activity. Exercise is essential for maintaining cardiovascular health, muscular strength, and mental clarity in addition to helping with weight management. Exercise options range from vigorous strength training and yoga to brisk walks, depending on one's physical level and interests. Establishing a program of exercise that you enjoy is essential to its sustainability.

Exercise has many physical advantages, but it's also a great way to manage stress and improve mental health. Exercise causes endorphins to be released, which lifts one's spirits and lowers anxiety. A weekly regimen that includes both aerobic and anaerobic activities guarantees a comprehensive approach to fitness, taking into account all facets of physical health.

## INTEGRATIVE THERAPIES

To address the mental, emotional, and spiritual aspects of health, integrative therapies combine traditional medical procedures with complementary methods.

Acupuncture, meditation, and massage therapy are among the practices that are becoming more and more well-known for their ability to enhance general well-being. To increase the effectiveness and lessen the negative effects of conventional medical treatments, these therapies are frequently utilized in addition to them.

Integrative therapies include mind-body techniques like yoga and mindfulness meditation as essential elements. By emphasizing the connection between physical and mental health, they promote a holistic view of wellness. Integrative therapies provide tools for stress management and self-care, enabling people to take an active role in their health journey.

## CONTROLLING TREATMENT SIDE EFFECTS

For people receiving medical care, controlling side effects is essential to preserving a high standard of living. The negative effects of radiation, chemotherapy, and other medical procedures might differ greatly. Collaboration with healthcare providers is crucial to create individualized symptom management plans.

Support from nutrition is crucial for reducing adverse effects. Changing to a diet that targets symptoms like nausea, exhaustion, or digestive problems, for example, can improve the body's resistance to treatment. Depending on a person's skills, physical activity can also help manage adverse effects like weariness and muscle weakness.

Integrative therapies, including acupuncture and meditation, can alleviate pain, anxiety, and other treatment-related issues in addition to conventional therapy. Creating a solid support network including friends, family, and support groups is also crucial for overcoming the psychological and emotional challenges associated with treatment. A more thorough and patient-centered approach to wellness during trying times is ensured by a multifaceted approach to side effect management.

## SURVIVORSHIP AND AFTERCARE FOLLOWING THERAPY

A crucial stage in the survivor journey is life after cancer treatment, which involves a variety of social, emotional, and physical adaptations. Many people experience a sense of relief as well as reflection upon finishing treatment, which marks the start of a new chapter in their survivorship and the end of a time dominated by medical interventions. It is important to understand that living after treatment does not always mean going back to exactly as things were before the diagnosis; instead, survivors frequently have to navigate a "new normal" that involves constant modifications to their physical and mental well-being as well as their way of life.

## KEEPING AN EYE OUT FOR RECURRENCE

Being vigilant for a possible cancer recurrence is an important part of life after treatment. A mix of self-awareness, routine medical checkups, and follow-up appointments is used to monitor for recurrence. It is advised that survivors stay aware of any changes in their bodies and notify their healthcare team right away if they have any concerns.

In the post-treatment phase, survivors learn to manage the uncertainties that come with recurrence worry, which is marked by a careful balancing act between optimism and vigilance. Maintaining a healthy lifestyle, which includes a balanced diet and frequent exercise, can improve general well-being and act as a preventative step for survivorship.

## RESCHEDULED APPOINTMENTS

Appointments for follow-up are essential to the continuum of care for survivors. These consultations have several functions, from keeping an eye on the patient's physical well-being to resolving any unresolved emotional or psychological issues. The purpose of routine medical checkups is to identify possible recurrences early on and enable prompt, if necessary, intervention.

Additionally, follow-up appointments give survivors a forum to voice any lingering worries, get advice on how to handle treatment side effects, and cultivate a feeling of continuous support from the medical staff.

# HONORING SIGNIFICANT OCCASIONS

A crucial component of the survivor journey is celebrating milestones, which stand for accomplishments and wins along the path. These benchmarks could take many different forms, such as finishing a specific time frame after treatment, reaching individual health objectives, or even getting back to your regular hobbies.

Festivities function as potent validations of fortitude and adaptability, strengthening the survivor's feeling of self-determination and achievement. In addition, they offer a chance for social interaction, as friends, family, and medical professionals come together to recognize and celebrate the survivor's journey.

Living after cancer treatment is a complex and dynamic experience that includes a range of well-being factors. A thorough survivorship framework incorporates the ideas of milestone celebration, follow-up checkups, and recurrence monitoring. Achieving this stage calls for striking a balance between proactive healthcare engagement, self-awareness, and acknowledging one's accomplishments. Being a survivor is not just about reaching a certain point; it's a continuous journey, and the help you receive during this time is essential to building resilience and encouraging a happy life after cancer.

# CHAPTER SEVEN

## AWARENESS AND ADVOCACY

### BECOMING YOUR ADVOCATE

In the healthcare industry and other spheres of life, the idea of becoming one's advocate is essential. It entails actively participating in the comprehension and maintenance of one's well-being. Being an advocate in the health setting entails actively taking part in decisions about medical care, available treatments, and general health management. This includes asking questions, sharing preferences and concerns with healthcare practitioners, and staying educated about one's health circumstances.

Being an empowered advocate is essential, particularly when dealing with intricate and subtle health issues like vaginal cancer. This proactive approach promotes a sense of control and autonomy over an individual's health journey in addition to guaranteeing the finest available care. It entails keeping up with the most recent advancements in medical research, getting second views, and fostering a cooperative relationship with medical specialists.

## INCREASING AWARENESS

Increasing awareness is a very effective way to deal with health problems, such as vaginal cancer. It entails educating the public, spreading knowledge, and dispelling myths and stigmas related to the illness. Reaching a wide audience is the goal of awareness programs, which also encourage proactive health-seeking habits by promoting empathy and understanding.

Increasing awareness is essential for early detection and prevention of vaginal cancer. Informing people about symptoms, risk factors, and screening alternatives can help in early diagnosis and better results. Awareness campaigns can also lessen the stigma attached to gynecological malignancies by fostering an honest conversation that supports a community that supports those who are impacted and their families.

Endorsing Research Initiatives for Vaginal Cancer: Research projects are critical to expanding our knowledge of vaginal cancer and creating more potent treatment alternatives. Contributions in kind, involvement in clinical trials, and lobbying for more money for research are all crucial elements of strengthening current initiatives in the sector. Research is essential for determining risk factors, investigating cutting-edge treatment options, and, in the end, enhancing prognosis for vaginal cancer patients.

## GETTING INTO CONTACT WITH ADVOCACY GROUPS

Getting involved with advocacy groups is a proactive approach to support the group's efforts to combat vaginal cancer. These groups are essential in bringing attention to the issue, offering assistance, and pushing for legislative reforms that will help those impacted by gynecological cancers. People can share their stories, raise awareness of their experiences, and advance a larger movement aimed at enhancing the prognosis and standard of living for vaginal cancer patients by actively engaging in advocacy activities.

A holistic approach to overcoming the issues faced by vaginal cancer involves becoming one's advocate, increasing awareness, funding research, and interacting with advocacy organizations. These deeds empower people, create a community of support, and advance continuous efforts to improve early detection, prevention, and treatment of this complicated health issue.